WE ARE
THE
LORD'S

WE ARE THE LORD'S

*A Catholic Guide to
Difficult End-of-Life Questions*

FR. JEFFREY KIRBY, STD

TAN Books
Charlotte, North Carolina

Cover design by Caroline K. Green

Library of Congress Control Number: 2019936355

ISBN: 978-1-5051-1461-4

Published in the United States by
TAN Books
PO Box 410487
Charlotte, NC 28241
www.TANBooks.com

Printed in the United States of America

To the venerable members of the Knights of Malta

Contents

Acknowledgments

I'd like to express my appreciation to *The Catholic Miscellany*, the diocesan newspaper of the Diocese of Charleston, for its permission to use various columns I've written for them over the years. Versions of these columns, often with greater or lesser revisions, appear throughout this book.

Thank you to Father Pau Agulles of the Holy Cross University in Rome. As my dissertation advisor during my doctoral research on the formation of consciences among medical personnel, he was the paradigm of patience and kindness as he provided both guidance and encouragement throughout the different phases of the research. Aspects of that research are found throughout this book, especially in chapter 2 on redemptive suffering.

I'm grateful to the Catholic Conference of South Carolina for its permission to use notes that I prepared for workshops with them on end-of-life care. Most of chapter 6 on the principles of discernment consists of these notes.

I'm also grateful to Crux Catholic Media who allowed me to use a portion of a previous column I wrote for them on praying for the dead in chapter 9.

Thank you to Jackie Gallagher, Dame of the Order of Malta, who made this entire project possible. It was Jackie's concern for people who are suffering, their families, and those loved ones who carry the cross of being medical proxies that brought this book from a passing idea into the book you're holding. Thank you, Jackie! May God bless your loving kindness to the sick and suffering and may Our Lady of Lourdes bless your service to those in need.

I'd like to also thank my nephew, Aaron Kirby, a law student in Alabama, who amidst his multiple other tasks helped me with the research and editing of the manuscript.

Introduction

The Help You Need

Are you in a dilemma and have to make a pressing end-of-life decision? Are you or a loved one in intense pain or in the dying process? Are you confused or emotionally drained and unsure of how to answer questions about medical treatment? If you find yourself in these situations, my heart goes out to you. This book was written specifically to help with the moral challenges that arise toward the end of life. I pray it brings you helpful information and a sense of peace and comfort during your most difficult moments.

Urgent Questions?

If you have urgent questions, please go directly to chapter 7 (page 44). There you will find a series of rapid questions and answers about specific medical issues that are meant to be a quick reference and help to those in pressing situations.

Principles and Guidance

If you have a little more time, please attempt to read through the whole book as each chapter develops and explains biblical wisdom and principles of discernment. These explanations can help expand your moral horizons and give you a strong outline from which you can discern moral questions and find holy and good answers.

Children of the Light

While we all die, the process of dying has never been particularly easy. The path of transitioning from this life to the next is a difficult one, but it doesn't have to be a distressing one. Distress is caused by uncertainty, which festers into dilemmas. But we were not made for such darkness. We are the children of God. We have been redeemed by Jesus Christ, who conquered death. The Holy Spirit dwells within us. And so, for the believer, *distress is overcome by truth*. The darkness of dilemma is scattered by light. We have been shown the way.

Divine Wisdom

The pages of this book, therefore, are drawn from divine wisdom, as contained in Sacred Tradition and in the Sacred Scriptures. This heavenly teaching has been given to us by our loving Father, who is well pleased with us. He sent us his Son, Jesus Christ, who accompanies us through life and death. The Lord Jesus desires to show us the fullness of life, as well as the path to a happy and holy death.

In order to be consistent with the light of divine wisdom, this book is written in complete fidelity to the teaching office, called the magisterium, of the Catholic

Church. It readily acknowledges the promise of the Lord Jesus upon his Church; namely, that it shall not err in matters relating to faith and morals.

On occasion, when the magisterium of the Catholic Church has not given a specific teaching on a moral question, then the book will acknowledge that neutrality (or on-going discernment) of the Church. After this indication, however, the book will seek to provide an opinion and explain it theologically.

Context and Perspective

As the author of this book, I write with the precision demanded of theology. I hold a doctorate in moral theology from the Holy Cross University in Rome, a Master of Arts in Philosophy from the Franciscan University of Steubenville, and a Masters in Bioethics from the Queen of Apostles Athenaeum in Rome. My writing, however, also reflects the compassion demanded of a loving shepherd. I'm currently the pastor of Our Lady of Grace Parish in Indian Land, South Carolina, and an adjunct professor of theology at Belmont Abbey College and at Pontifex University. These pastoral positions help me to accompany people in their sufferings and in the dilemmas of life and death.

Of course, theological teachings and pastoral practice complement each other. They're two sides of the same coin. The heart softens the mind, while the mind elevates the heart. In life, we need both. This book seeks to provide insights for each.

And so, let's begin.

CHAPTER 1

Life as a Gift

Death Is Not the End

If you read the introduction, you might've noticed the last words were, "let's begin." While that might seem like a strange choice of words for a book about end-of-life decisions, it's actually a fitting play on words since death is not an end but a beginning. Death is the start of a new journey. So . . . let's begin.

No Person Is a Burden

Oftentimes in dealing with those who are terminally ill, or those who are facing long-term medical treatment, I've heard them say, "I don't want to be a burden to my children!" Trying to break the tension, I'll often reply, "You're too late! You've been a burden to them since the day they were born!"

The comment usually provokes a laugh or a confused look. But the point is made. Love is filled with burdens. Relationships are overflowing with burdens. Saint Paul tells us, "Bear one another's burdens, and so fulfil the law of Christ" (Gal 6:2).

It's true that the term "burden" can be applied to love and relationships, but it's also true—and we have to be careful of this distinction—that it should never be applied to a person. People are not burdens. Each of us are made in the image and likeness of God (cf. Gn 1:26–28). Simply put, God is our Father and we look like him. This identity bestows on all of us an inalienable dignity that must be respected and cherished, even in the midst of the burdens and exhaustion that are a part of giving care (or receiving it).

This basic point has to be made since we live in a culture intoxicated with utilitarianism, which is the belief that value is only found in what we can receive or in what we can get from someone else. We live in a culture that has taught people that any inconvenience for another person, or any service that makes us uncomfortable, is unmerited. We're told that the recipient of such care is a burden, especially those who are the most vulnerable and weak among us. Many in our culture have bought this lie.

In contrast to our society's utilitarianism, Christian teaching has always asserted that the only adequate response to a person is love (cf. Jn 13:34–35). By focusing on love—seeking the good in others—we can expose selfishness that disguises itself as compassion. We can break a downward spiral that overemphasizes the hardship of loved ones to the neglect of the person who is principally suffering. And so it is true love for another, made in God's image, that helps us see the person's dignity. This realization calls us to order our own emotions and difficulties according to the other person's dignity. It liberates us from self-absorption and helps us see the good that is being done and the beauty that is being defended.

The Image of God

For the Christian believer, creation is the foundation of God's saving work, which is fulfilled in Jesus Christ. Redemption happens because we exist. The world was created for our good and we were created because of God's love for us. This point is worth stressing: we are not a *something* but a *someone*, and we only exist because God loves us. If God ceased to love us, we would completely disappear, not existing and never having existed. All that we are, including our history, home, and health, dwells in existence because of God's love.

The living God seals his love for us by placing his very own image and likeness within us. Unlike the angels or the animals, we bear a special mark that identifies us as the sons and daughters of God. We are consecrated and dedicated to him and his glory. Our lives are temples of his majesty and witnesses to his care for creation. The image that we each bear is a singular narrative all its own. No one else can repeat or duplicate who we are. No one else can reveal what we can disclose about God since the image we have of him is unrepeatable (cf. Ps 8:4–8).

Understood in this light, the Christian is comfortable acknowledging that every human life is a true gift from God. Life is the first and highest of all gifts since it is the means by which all other gifts are received. But life is also a fragile gift, entrusted to the person who receives it, to his family and community, and to the entire human race. Life, therefore, is a gift that is also a sacred responsibility.

Body and Soul

As human beings made in God's image, we consist of a body and a soul. Both our bodies and our souls share in the image of God.

The body is not to be diminished, dismissed as some raw matter with no identity, or merely seen as a vehicle that carries our souls around. No, the body shares in our dignity. It must be respected, cared for, and properly esteemed. Our souls should not be approached as somehow our "true selves," as if the body was a foreign component to our personhood. Such a false view has rationalized all sorts of medical neglect, disordered compassion, calculated harm, and willful manipulation of our bodies.

The complementarity of our souls and bodies are reflected in many ways, especially when we love, express delight, give thanks, and suffer. For example, our souls share in the sufferings of our bodies and vice versa. If our body has a high temperature, then our will is weakened and virtue is more difficult. If our souls are clouded with melancholy, then our bodies experience a weakening of muscle capacity.

In discerning medical treatment and care, therefore, we have to be cautious not to isolate the soul from the body, or the body from the soul. As human beings, we are both body and soul and the care we give ourselves, or receive from others, must consider both these portions of our personhood.

Quality of Life

Given our identity as human persons and our existential connection to God, we have to understand that our self-possession, popularly called autonomy, is not an absolute power. Our autonomy is dependent. It has to make reference to God and his providential design of our bodies and souls, as well as his divine law and the family and community to which he has entrusted us.

Our autonomy, therefore, should never be viewed as independent from our dignity as children of God. Our definition of "quality of life" is not simply the power to live however we want in whatever way we want. Seen holistically and in light of our transcendence as the children of God, our quality of life is grounded upon our dignity. It is matured by love and an openness to live with inconvenience, discomfort, imperfection, and suffering. Our quality of life is improved through a willingness to surrender what we prefer for the sake of what is good and in accord with our dignity as the children of God.

Conclusion

The realization of our esteemed place in God's creation, and of our dignity as his beloved sons and daughters, is the first and fundamental principle for us in evaluating medical care and treatment. All our decisions must be based upon and flow from the reality that we are a human person, with a body and soul, made in God's image.

Our acceptance of this dignity frees us from isolation and self-absorption. It helps us to place our autonomy within our relationship with God, our neighbor, and the world around us. Our dignity shows us that we are not sovereign selves but people united to God and to other people. And so we are not only beholden to ourselves but also to our Creator and to others.

CHAPTER 2

Redemptive Suffering

Original Justice

Christian teaching recounts that the human family was created by God in a state of perfect justice marked by harmony between a person's soul and body, among human persons in a community, and between humanity and the rest of the created world. Within the human person, the soul held mastery over the body, and both the body and soul shared an inheritance of eternal life.

Our Rebellion and Its Consequences

Our first parents were given this blessed state and were told not to eat the fruit of the Tree of the Knowledge of Good and Evil (cf. Gn 2:17). This directive was to show humanity its need for God and its responsibility to acknowledge God as both its Creator as well as the Author of the laws that govern all things, including the moral law of right and wrong. The parents of humanity, however, chose to rebel against their loving Creator and chose a path contrary to the one indicated by him. Adam and Eve abused the freedom that was given to them to love God by choosing a love of self. They introduced discord between themselves and God, within their own personhood and between each other, and with the world around them.

The prohibition given by God was against a willed attempt to legislate and determine what is right and wrong for oneself. It was the renunciation of the sovereign self, seeing itself as the only source of law, removing itself from God, community, and the world, and then deciding in its own isolation what is right and wrong.

As a consequence of the disobedience of humanity's first parents, human nature itself and all creation fell from grace. The soul lost its own internal harmony and the mastery it held over the body. While created good, the human person would now have an inclination toward evil and darkness. Consequently, human persons are inclined to their own comfort or interests over those of their neighbors, and humanity sees the world as a means of conquest and profit rather than a place calling for care and stewardship. Ever since the Fall, the ability to believe and discern moral goodness through the natural light of reason has become more difficult and strenuous for humanity.

Suffering and Illness

With the soul's mastery over the body lost, the human body would now experience death. The human person would suffer the plight of having an immortal soul within a mortal body. And with the loss of beatitude and the immortality of the body, suffering and illness became a part of human life.

Pope John Paul II wrote the apostolic letter *Salvifici Doloris* on suffering after his attempted assassination and the long series of hospital visits and medical procedures that were required to restore him to health. In this letter, he wrote, "Man suffers on account of evil, which is a certain lack, limitation or distortion of good. We could say that man suffers because of a good in which he does not share, from which in a certain sense he is cut off, or of which he has deprived himself. He particularly suffers when he 'ought'—in the normal order of things—to have a share in this good and does not have it."[1]

Christian belief, therefore, sees suffering and illness within the theological context of the fall from grace and acknowledges them as evils within human life. They are not seen as the consequences of the actual sins of any one person after the Fall but as a dark inheritance from the original sin of our first parents and the subsequent fall within human nature itself. From the Fall, human history will include the sorrow and drama of illness and suffering. The human story is marked by questions about evil, inquiries about suffering, debates over human dignity and quality of life, medical battles against illness and the care of the sick, and struggles with faith and understanding about moral goodness and responsibility. For the Christian believer and the discerning person of good

---

1   Pope John Paul II, apostolic letter *Salvifici Doloris*, no. 7.

will, answers to these questions begin with the Fall; it is the source and cause of human suffering and illness.

But do these evils have the last word in the human experience? Is there possibly a deeper understanding of suffering available to the human family? Let's find out.

Light of the World

In the fallenness of humanity, God the Son came as the Light of the World. When the Son of God came, was it as a removed figure falling from the skies? Was he born from the mind of his divine Father or from a peculiar sexual encounter, as was commonly said of divinities within the myths of Greece and Rome? Was the Son of God a ghost or a theophany of some sort that merely appeared to be human?

Let's be perfectly clear: the Second Person of the Holy Trinity came as a human being. As St. Paul taught, "But when the time had fully come, God sent forth his Son, born of woman, born under the law, to redeem those who were under the law, so that we might receive adoption as sons" (Gal 4:4–5).

The divine Son became a full human being and experienced all things truly human. He showed humanity its dignity as the children of God and taught the human family how it is to live. The Second Person of the Holy Trinity took on human flesh in Jesus of Nazareth. He came as the fullness of all God's revelation. In summary, all that humanity had discerned of God through the light of natural reason and all that was supernaturally revealed to humanity about God was recapitulated and fulfilled in Jesus Christ.

What was Jesus Christ's work within the human family? How is his ministry to be understood? What was the light he brought to humanity? How can the medical community benefit from his saving work and witness?

Fully Human and Privation of Being

Jesus Christ was true God and true Man. As such, he was the model of what it means to be human. In his life and work, the Lord Jesus showed humanity how we are to live and serve others. By understanding the human identity of Jesus Christ, humanity (and the medical community) can see a brighter reflection of humanity and can better and more deeply hear and appreciate the Lord's teachings and witness among us.

The Lord Jesus does not teach as an outsider but as a human being, as someone within the human family. In comprehending Jesus Christ in this way, humanity can more deeply understand its own goodness and dignity. The human person's own identity as someone—not a "something"—with an incommunicable dimension that is made for self-donation and community life can be seen with clearer eyes in Christ. Both of these truths are reflected in the mystery of the Holy Trinity and in Jesus's ministry.

But what about the fallenness of humanity? Don't the sins of humanity prove that it cannot follow the example given by Jesus Christ? Doesn't sin show that humanity is only motivated by ambition and the desire for pleasure?

How is sin to be understood in light of the ministry of Jesus Christ?

Humanity can easily see our fallenness. From concentration camps and killing fields to racism and religious extremism to the abuse of medicine or the neglect of those who are suffering, we could easily come to believe that human persons are evil. Left to itself, such a conclusion about humanity would be understandable (even if wrong). Sin, however, has always been understood as a privation of being. In seeing that the world and the human person are good and have a natural orientation to goodness (although heavily influenced by an impulse to evil), sin is seen as a privation—a lacking or removal of being—and something that takes away goodness.

In seeing sin as this privation, we understand that sin and evil are not portions of creation and humanity. When, therefore, it is said that Jesus Christ was fully human and yet lacking in sin, it reflects the reality that sin is not human or real but is actually anti-human and anti-reality. Sin, therefore, does not have the power to define humanity, even as it takes away the richness of the human essence and veils the goodness of the person and of creation, covering them with darkness.

As the exemplar of humanity, Jesus Christ is without sin and he shows us how to live as fully human beings. As the Savior of humanity and the source of reconciliation between God and Man, Jesus Christ takes away the sins of humanity, allowing the person to be free to live out his inheritance as a person and a child of God. Humanity, therefore, is defined by goodness and love.

As Pope St. John Paul II taught at the World Youth Day in Toronto in 2002: "We are not the sum of our weaknesses and failures. We are the sum of the Father's love for us and our real capacity to become the image of his Son."

If the Lord Jesus did not sin or experience sin, how can he be the exemplar of humanity? How can someone without sin attempt to understand human life that has been marred by sin and guilt? How can someone without sin be a source of guidance to the medical community that finds itself in a diversity of situations and must attempt to discern the best course of action for those who are ill or suffering? What credibility does Jesus Christ have to humanity and to the medical community?

The Capacity to Suffer

In our attempt to understand sin, it must be placed within its proper conclusion as a privation of being. Humanity cannot allow itself to be defined by sin, which is a privation of goodness, or to allow sin to become a standard of maturation or wisdom. The human person is defined by goodness and virtue, and human maturity is given by love and through self-donation.

With this emphasis made, however, sin and guilt weigh heavily in the experiences of human life (as well as within medical practice and bioethical discernment). How, then, can the life and teachings of Jesus Christ help humanity? If Jesus is without sin, can he understand humanity and its struggles? How can Jesus's self-donation be appreciated and imitated within the human experience? In the end, what credibility does Jesus legitimately have toward humanity and the medical community?

In teaching that Jesus had a human soul as a part of his human nature, the Church acknowledges that he had a capacity to suffer and feel pain. Without a human soul, this experience would not have been possible. So when it is said that the Lord Jesus had no sin, it does not mean that he did not experience sin and its consequences in our world. As seen throughout the account of his life in the Gospels, we see that the Lord Jesus did experience mourning, tiredness, righteous anger, loss, distress, anxiety, agony, and fear of death and suffering, as well as other emotions and states within the human soul. Christ knows every experience and has felt every emotion of one who is suffering, as well as the empathy and compassion of the medical professional and the loved ones of those who are ill or suffering.

But does Jesus only remain in the spiritual and emotional aspects of suffering? What does he do with his knowledge and experience of human life and suffering? What example does he present to all people of good will? What does he model for the medical professional?

Salvation Through Suffering

No discussion of human life, or the practice of medicine, would be complete without addressing the full array of suffering, not only within the soul, but also in the body. In experiencing the fullness of human life, Jesus Christ understood and accepted all forms of suffering, and he desires to teach humanity (including the medical professional) the scope and truths surrounding human suffering.

As we saw, since humanity's fall from grace, suffering has been an evil within human life. Christian theology has always seen suffering as an evil and as a consequence of the original sin of Adam and Eve. In taking on our human nature, Jesus Christ accepted the suffering of humanity, *both* body and soul. From his life of poverty to living as a refugee in a foreign land to being hunted down as a criminal to the frustration of learning a trade to the death of his foster father to his experience of fatigue and thirst to being misunderstood, rejected, and unloved. All of his sufferings culminated in the cruelty and torture of his passion and the humiliation and asphyxiation of his death. In all these sufferings, he chose to accept, enter, and use suffering, which has been such a pivotal dilemma and source of anguish in human history, as the very means to manifest his love and self-donation for humanity. *Suffering itself would become the instrument of salvation.*

How is this possible? How did Jesus Christ use suffering for the redemption and renewal of humanity?

In taking on human suffering, the Lord Jesus went directly to sin, understood as the source of suffering in human life. In order to take away sin and vanquish its control on humanity, Jesus Christ became sin itself. He sought to destroy this privation of being, and its consequences of suffering and death, from the inside out. In becoming sin, Jesus Christ took upon himself all the sins of humanity throughout time. He endured the totality of human guilt, shame, alienation, grief, confusion, and the full panorama of darkness caused by sin.

The crucible for this radically human endeavor was the Lord's passion, which began in the Garden of Gethsemane. In the garden, as he took upon himself the sins of humanity, the Lord Jesus sweated blood, felt the full isolation caused by sin, and could not raise his eyes to the heavens. In the Garden of Gethsemane and by the full weight of his passion, death, and resurrection, Jesus proved his association with suffering humanity and began his passion, which would ultimately destroy the power of sin and death.

On account therefore of the unique depth of his human experience, Jesus Christ—true God and true Man—has complete credibility as the exemplar of what it means to be human. Additionally, his singular experiential knowledge of suffering in soul and body makes him the standard by which both the care of the sick and suffering can be evaluated and its moral discernment measured.

But if Jesus Christ has destroyed sin, why does illness and suffering still afflict humanity? How is humanity (and the medical community) to understand suffering in light of the ministry of Jesus Christ?

Redemptive Suffering

And now we come to the heart of this chapter. Everything up to this point was given as a foundation for us to fully understand redemptive suffering.

We must understand that while the ministry of Jesus Christ has destroyed the kingdom of sin and death, the consequences of sin still remain in the human experience. The difference, however, is that suffering—while an evil caused by original sin—can now become redemptive for the person and the community. Rather than seeing suffering in merely negative terms, the example and ministry of Jesus Christ now shows the human family a positive way in which suffering can be seen and accepted in human life.

Now, in Jesus Christ, suffering can be a source of repentance, purification, goodness, penance, renewal, hope, and empathy to others who are sick or suffering in some way. In the Lord Jesus, who offered his sufferings as a self-oblation and as a means of selfless service, humanity can see suffering as a new way of service to others and as a new means of self-donation and salvation for themselves and the whole world.

Conclusion

In the midst of bioethical discernment and the evaluation of medical procedures and treatments, we must understand the cause of suffering and its possible redemptive aspects. While not sought for its own good, we accept that suffering can bring about a greater good by the grace of God.

Inspired and enabled by Jesus Christ, the Christian believer is willing to accept pain and suffering so as to participate in the life and redemptive work of the Lord.

As believers, we must not waste our suffering but constantly see it in light of the Lord's own passion and death so that we can share in the glory of his resurrection (and be a means for others to also share in his glory).

CHAPTER 3

Dying With Dignity

The Dying Process

Some years ago, when a beloved mentor of mine was terminally ill, I asked him what it was like to prepare for death. He told me it was lonely.

I was surprised by his response because he was always surrounded by family, friends, and former students. When I asked him about his loneliness, he told me that the dying process is so unique that few could understand it. He said that his only source of consolation was his faith in Jesus Christ and the sure knowledge that the Lord was with him and understood what he was going through, even when no one else was able to fully understand.

This story illustrates that death is truly humanity's question, and it can be a purifying one. At different times, we all think about death, and at other times, we all seek to avoid it. Since everyone will die, the enduring inquiries about dying, death, and the afterlife continue to provoke curiosity, fear, and hope within the human family.

These are our questions because they touch our lives, and because of their gravity, these questions deserve attention and some strong resolutions within us.

What is death? What is meant by the dying process? Is there an afterlife? When all is said and done, in whom do I place my trust?

The conclusions we reach on these final questions will shape and help determine the way we live and interact with life and its joys and difficulties. They will actively influence the way we approach the dying process. In approaching these questions, will we allow them to be answered by our identity as the sons and daughters of God? Will we allow our faith in Jesus Christ to provide us a verified answer?

Perennial wisdom teaches us that we die as we live. My mentor was a man of faith. In his last days, his Christian faith provided answers to his questions, and that gave him tremendous and true consolation. As he had lived his entire life in Jesus Christ, so he died (and rose) in Jesus Christ.

In many respects, death is a contradiction to the life we lead now. It's at odds with our will to live. It relativizes our freedom, which our culture cherishes above all things. And so, as death will come for each human person, what will our answers be to the questions that surround it?

Another Example

A few years ago, a friend told me that he wasn't afraid of death. I was pretty impressed until he told me that he was just afraid of dying. I had to laugh. The idea of separating death from dying sounds comical, but there's actually some depth in the distinction.

Perhaps this friend is like most of us. The idea of being dead doesn't bother us (after all, we'll be dead), but the idea of dying can rattle our nerves. The experience is similar to a person who likes to go to foreign places but hates to travel!

As the intermediate process, dying has many of us unsettled. As a human reality, the dying process is our most extreme time of transition. We move from one well-known stage of life to a veiled, mysterious one. It is a time of understandable difficulty, of questions to our faith, sometimes of great pain, and a suffering of the heart as we have to give farewells to the people we love.

Fear of Dying

The stark reality of death can oftentimes scare us or lead us to see death merely as a terrible evil that must be avoided at all costs. The idea of losing our autonomy, our control over ourselves and our lives, makes us profoundly restless and agitated. The idea of permanently letting go of everything we have and of everyone that we love can terrify us. Within the forum of this restlessness and anxiety, we have to answer our questions.

If we place our trust in the Lord Jesus, we see that death has lost its sting (cf. 1 Cor 15:55–57). We unmask the lies surrounding death, and hope destroys all our fears. In the midst of this internal wrestling, we are reminded of our identity in Jesus Christ. In Christ, we are able to see the full reality of human existence, during and after this life.

St. Paul clearly teaches us that in life and in death, "we are the Lord's" (Rom 14:8).

In Christ, we see that our lives are a journey, and death is a process. And while death and dying may be difficult, the Lord Jesus can remove our anxieties. Death does not need to be an ultimate end or final goodbye.

If we allow him, the Lord will claim us as his own. By the power of his resurrection, death becomes a transition that only initiates a new phase of life, one that leads us from glory unto glory (cf. 2 Cor 3:18).

Our discipleship, with all its triumphs and failures throughout our lives, does not end in the dying process but is empowered and intensified through it. As in life, so in death, we are called to cling to the Lord Jesus, truly risen from the dead, and give him all the fears and struggles of our passing.

In turning to Jesus Christ, we realize that we are not alone. Jesus, our Good Shepherd, is with us. We are invited to give the end of our earthly lives to him, praying, "Into your hands, O Lord, I commend my spirit." Our faith encourages us in this radical act of faith. It offers us the sacramental presence of Jesus and echoes to all believers in every age the summons to die well in the Lord.

In this solemn responsibility that we have as believers in Jesus Christ, the Church walks with us and gives us clear and compassionate teachings to the various medical procedures and questions surrounding the dying process. Whether it is the use of breathing tubes, the continuation of nutrition and hydration, or the use of pain medication and palliative care, the Church offers us the teachings and wisdom of Jesus Christ so that we can die well and full in the abundance of his grace (or help a loved one do so).

We are called, therefore, to give our dying process—and all the decisions surrounding it—to the Lord Jesus. It is our last earthly gift to our loving Savior.

Dying With Dignity

In accompanying many people in the dying process who stand in different places in their relationship with God and the Lord Jesus, I have heard many people say, "I just want to die with dignity." The concept of dignity has become a crucible in the fear of dying. Many people are afraid of the unknown, worried about feeding tubes and fearful of being kept alive by machines. This uneasiness culminates in a misplaced concept of "dying with dignity."

Dying is a reality. We will all approach this process in one way or another. As addressed in this chapter, there is an understandable and natural fear of dying. Faith and its truths, however, can help us address and temper this fear by God's grace.

In addressing the fear of dying, we must also address dignity. As discussed in chapter 1, dignity is given to us by God, and we have to apply this understanding of dignity to our dying process. As emphasized, our dignity is not given to us by our parents or by the government or insurance companies. Our dignity is not even given to us by ourselves or our health, utility, or a supposed quality of life. Our dignity is given to us by our Creator, and so nothing, and no one, can take it from us.

And so, in response to people who fearfully say, "I want to die with dignity," I say confidently, "I have good news! You *will* die with dignity. Nothing can take your dignity from you. In whatever way you die, and whatever might happen to you in the process, the God who created you and gave you your dignity will be the God who walks with you and gives you the strength to die a good death in his grace. You can trust him!"

Conclusions

In the process of dying (or of watching a loved one die), we have to be aware of the influence and flurry caused by fear. Whether it's a fear of diminished capacity, or losing our control, or being kept alive in ways we would not prefer, such fear can be matured, enlightened, and consoled by the truths given by Jesus Christ.

The truths of faith attested to by the passion, death, and resurrection of Jesus Christ provide us with firm and substantiated answers to our questions about death. These truths call us to a greater reliance on the Lord, especially in our uncertainty and pain. It is this very reliance that helps us place our autonomy within our relationship with the Lord. It guides us to a greater realization of our dignity as the children of God, a dignity which cannot be taken away by anything of this world.

CHAPTER 4

Saved by Hope

Are You Saved?

One summer as a college student working at a department store, I was approached during my lunch break by a coworker. He sat down next to me and innocently asked, "Have you been saved?"

Before I realized what he was asking me, I thought, "Saved from what?" Eventually, I understood what he was asking. I had heard the question before but was just taken off guard by being asked the question at work.

In South Carolina and throughout the Bible Belt, Catholics have become pretty accustomed to being asked such a surprising question. In many social environments, we have almost come to expect the question from friends, neighbors, and even coworkers. In preparation for the question, or perhaps for our own spiritual growth, we should ask ourselves: have I been saved? What does that really mean?

Saved by Hope

As we reflect on the many questions around death and the medical care and treatment that surround it, it's important for us to see things in the full light of eternity. As believers, our entire way of life depends on our belief in the Lord's care for us, manifested most powerfully in his glorious resurrection through which he calls us to live with him in eternity. This understanding of God's goodness and our invitation to live forever in heaven raise some serious questions about our salvation. How do we answer them? How are we saved?

The Gospels teach us that salvation from darkness and its consequences, and the reward of eternal life in heaven, are found in Jesus Christ. In our baptism and the acceptance of his Lordship in our lives, we find hope for this salvation. St. Paul reminds us that we are "saved in hope." He writes, "We know that the whole creation has been groaning with labor pains together until now; and not only the creation, but we ourselves, who have the first fruits of the Spirit, groan inwardly as we wait for adoption as sons, the redemption of our bodies. For in this hope we were saved" (Rom 8:22–24).

Since it is at the heart of our understanding of salvation, it is very important for us to understand the biblical notion of hope, which has become a distorted and abused virtue in our society. It's worth clarifying this virtue and showing why it's so important in the Christian way of life.

For Christians, hope is always placed in God. We do not hope in ourselves without God, or in human efforts without God's presence. To do so would be to use hope as a disguise for pride and arrogance. Christians are called to understand that salvation comes from hoping in the

Lord and in his divine providence, which is his care for us in this life and his welcoming of us into eternal life.

Hope is placing a profound trust of our life, existence, and well-being in the hands of God. It is trusting him unconditionally and actively nurturing in ourselves "eyes of faith," which helps us see his work among us and helps us eagerly long to be with him forever in heaven.

Our hope in God can help us appreciate the blessings and sorrows of this life. It places them all within a beautiful mosaic of God's love and care for us. Hope heals our wounds and lifts up our spirits. It strengthens our faith and empowers our ability to love. Hope teaches us to place an appropriate trust in our loved ones and in the good things of this world.

By hoping in God, we rely completely and ultimately on him, especially when we are weak or experiencing pain and suffering. In this radical hope, in spite of the world's darkness and brokenness, we find an assurance of God's promises, the power to believe and cooperate with his grace, and the openness that is needed to let the Lord change us for the better and make us fit for the kingdom of God.

In hope, we are *being saved* in Jesus Christ. We hope to one day share eternal life with him.

Conclusion

We know as believers that our dignity comes from God. We know that we've been given a unique identity as his sons and daughters. We readily place our autonomy within the Lord's divine providence, which is his care for us in this life. This trust builds up hope in us. Hope allows us to place everything, even suffering and anguish, within the light of eternity.

It is the hope of heaven that strengthens us and refocuses us when pain or turmoil seek to distract us. It is the hope of eternal life that calls us back to an obedience of faith and to the firm desire to give ourselves, and our dying process, to the Lord.

Hope reminds us that the suspension of suffering or the conclusion of pain in this life are not our final goals and that even these, as beneficial as they can be, must be placed within divine wisdom and must cooperate with the workings of grace which labor to make us fit for eternal life with God.

CHAPTER 5

Judgment Before God

A Better Place?

After our dying process and death, we will all stand before the judgment seat of God. Admittedly, the reality of God's judgment after our death is an uncomfortable subject. It's a topic that many in our society would prefer to avoid or outright deny in one way or another. The notion of being judged for the lives we've lived and to receive an eternal, unstoppable, reward or condemnation is an overwhelming reality for most people who live in a culture saturated by a licentious freedom and a radical notion of personal autonomy.

With this backdrop, we can observe a few predominant responses in our culture. For example, we regularly hear, "He's going to a better place." It appears that even heaven itself is being replaced by the assurance of this "better place." In this presumption, the possibility of hell is rejected, and we are told that the only thing necessary for us to reach this better place is that we die. Death becomes the only condition for an undefined eternal bliss. The underlying belief in this trend is that all dead people deserve and are in this better place.

Made Fit for the Kingdom

Our lives, and the way we use our free will, are far too significant for such an empty system of beliefs. Our capacity for greatness and holiness is not adequately acknowledged in this generic system. And the temptation toward evil and maliciousness is too serious a reality to smooth over and normalize it.

Where are Jesus and the biblical notions of judgment, heaven, and hell in these cultural expressions? Where is love and our call to holiness? Where is our faith and hope?

If eternal salvation was as superficial as some believe, why did God become a man and die on the cross?

In drawing close to the Lord Jesus, we should ask the pressing question, voiced in the Gospel by the rich young man: "What shall I do to inherit eternal life?" (Lk 18:18).

This revealing question cuts through human presumption on one side and despair on the other. The Lord gives an initial answer to the question, telling us simply, "Follow the Commandments."

In his public ministry, Jesus repeatedly announces that he has come to make us "fit" for the kingdom of God. The Commandments are our first teachers, and they prepare our hearts for virtue and the deeper workings of God's grace. In this opportunity given to us by Jesus, we each have the task of "working out" our salvation. We aspire to become better people after God's own heart.

As we follow the Commandments, love summons more from us. Jesus eventually says to each of us, "Sell what you have . . . and come, follow me" (Mk 10:21). We are called to give everything to Jesus and seek to be completely transformed by his grace.

In this process, we change as persons: humility tempers pride, forgiveness heals retribution, kindness disintegrates anger, and we begin to see the visible signs which teach us about heaven. We know that we are being made fit to live in that kingdom. This is our task in life, and this is why God became a man and died and rose for us.

Conclusions

As human beings made in God's image, we live forever. But where we will live in eternity is determined *now*. We will die and live eternally as we have lived in this earthly life. If pride, lust, anger, envy, and the kingdom of sin and darkness have ruled our hearts, and we do not seek the help of God, then the pattern will continue, and we will live eternally in that wayward kingdom, which is called hell.

If, however, we draw close to Jesus and, in the failures and successes of our discipleship, we hope in him and try to cooperate with his grace and be transformed into better people, then the pattern will continue and we will live in that kingdom of light which we sought in our earthly lives. We will live forever in heaven.

CHAPTER 6

Principles of Discernment

The Obedience of Faith

The question of bioethics and end-of-life directives affects the lives of every person. People of good will seek to make end-of-life decisions based on their discernment of the natural moral law, their own moral sense, and their understanding of benefits, burdens, rights, and responsibilities.

Christian believers are called to this same process of discernment but are greatly aided by the teachings of Jesus Christ and his Church. As disciples of the Lord Jesus, we declare that our lives are not our own: "For to me to live is Christ" (Phil 1:21). And so we are called to give the "obedience of faith" (cf. Rom 1:5; 16:26) throughout our lives, which includes the dying process.

Pope St. John Paul II explained faith in this way:

> It is urgent to rediscover and to set forth once more the authentic reality of the Christian faith, which is not simply a set of propositions to be accepted with intellectual assent.
>
> Rather, faith is a lived knowledge of Christ, a

living remembrance of his commandments, and a truth to be lived out. A word, in any event, is not truly received until it passes into action, until it is put into practice.

Faith is a decision involving one's whole existence. It is an encounter, a dialogue, a communion of love and of life between the believer and Jesus Christ, the Way, and the Truth, and the Life (cf. Jn 14:6). It entails an act of trusting abandonment to Christ, which enables us to live as he lived (cf. Gal 2:20), in profound love of God and of our brothers and sisters.[2]

The Rich Young Man

With the above in mind, let's discuss some principles from which we can ground our end-of-life discernment in. The best place to do this, of course, is Sacred Scripture. We can go to the story of the rich young man and use this story to elucidate central principles of discernment for the Christian believer:

> And behold, one came up to him, saying, "Teacher, what good deed must I do, to have eternal life?" And he said to him, "Why do you ask me about what is good? One there is who is good. If you would enter life, keep the commandments." He said to him, "Which?" And Jesus said, "You shall not kill, You shall not commit adultery, You shall not steal, You

---

2   Pope John Paul II, *Veritatis Splendor*, no. 88.

shall not bear false witness Honor your father and
mother, and, You shall love your neighbor as yourself." The young man said to him, "All these I have
observed; what do I still lack?" Jesus said to him,
"If you would be perfect, go, sell what you possess
and give to the poor, and you will have treasure in
heaven; and come, follow me." (Mt 19:16–21)

This young man has stepped out of the crowd and
approached Jesus, seeking an answer to a most important
question.

What was that question? Pope St. John Paul II helps
us figure that out:

In the young man, whom Matthew's Gospel does
not name, we can recognize every person who, con-
sciously or not, approaches Christ the Redeemer of
man and questions him about morality.

For the young man, the question is not so
much about rules to be followed, but about the full
meaning of life.

This is in fact the aspiration at the heart of
every human decision and action, the quiet search-
ing and interior prompting which sets freedom in
motion. This question is ultimately an appeal to the
absolute Good which attracts us and beckons us; it
is the echo of a call from God who is the origin and
goal of man's life.[3]

---

3   Ibid., no. 7.

First Principle of Discerning End-of-Life Questions: Objective Moral Order and Our Dignity

Let's examine the conversation between Jesus and the rich young man a little more so that we can discern a few key principles in how we go about making end-of-life decisions.

Having approached Jesus, the rich young man asks a revealing question: "Teacher, what good must I do to have eternal life?" The inquiry indicates an acknowledgment of eternity and of heaven. It shows his sincere desire when he asks, "What must I do," as well as an acceptance of an objective criteria outside of himself. The young man cannot give the answer to himself. The answer is not solely within him. He must look beyond his own world, his own confusion, his own suffering, and ultimately beyond his own desire.

Again Pope St. John Paul II teaches, "The question which the rich young man puts to Jesus of Nazareth is one which rises from the depths of his heart. It is an essential and unavoidable question for the life of every man, for it is about the moral good which must be done, and about eternal life. The young man senses that there is a connection between moral good and the fulfilment of his own destiny.[4]

In the exchange, the Lord Jesus responds to the use of the term "good" by the rich young man. He indicates that the answer to his question can only be found in the One

---

4   Ibid., no. 8.

who is good; namely, in the Creator. The Lord is pointing the rich young man to the things that are above him. But he misses it.

We hear again from the saintly John Paul II:

> To ask about the good, in fact, ultimately means to turn towards God, the fullness of goodness.
>
> Jesus shows that the young man's question is really a religious question, and that the goodness that attracts and at the same time obliges man has its source in God, and indeed is God himself.
>
> God alone is worthy of being loved "with all one's heart, and with all one's soul, and with all one's mind" (Mt 22:37). He is the source of man's happiness.
>
> Jesus brings the question about morally good action back to its religious foundations, to the acknowledgment of God, who alone is goodness, fullness of life, the final end of human activity, and perfect happiness.[5]

And so our first principle of discernment is the recognition of our Creator and, more immediately, the objective order of moral truth beyond us.

It is "objective" in that it is beyond the subject, which is our own person. It's beyond us because we didn't create it, we can't change it (without moral peril), and if we want a good decision, one that brings peace, we must discern and decide according to it.

---

5   Ibid., no. 9.

One example of this objective truth is our dignity. In making end-of-life decisions, some will say, "But I just want to die with dignity." And they will. We all do. As we saw in a previous chapter, our dignity is not given by our health, autonomy, laws or government, or even by ourselves. Our dignity is given to us by our Creator. It is inalienable. No one, no thing, can take it away. Therefore, this inalienable dignity demands respect. It is the foundation of our human vocation, our call to live as full human beings, cherishing, respecting, and flourishing within our own dignity and that of others.

This means that in terms of end-of-life planning, while we must discern many things in the realm of treatment, we have boundaries. Our personal will, or the desire for autonomy, are not sovereign. These must be placed within our human dignity and the objective order of moral goodness, which is binding on all people of good will (and is seen as a manifestation of God's will by believers). This shows us that we cannot take our own lives or cause willful harm to our well-being.

But from here, the conversation between Jesus and the rich young man continues.

Second Principle of Discerning End-of-Life Questions: Our Specific Vocation

In the exchange, the Lord Jesus emphasizes the objective order of life by summarizing the Ten Commandments.

And Pope John Paul II explains, "The moral life presents itself as the response due to the many gratuitous

initiatives taken by God out of love for man."⁶ The Rich
Young Man claims to have followed the commandments
since his youth and so asks, "What still do I lack?" (Mt
19:20).

This second question points not only to our human
vocation (described earlier) but also to our particular vocation; namely, to our specific place and mission
in the plan of salvation. While the commandments are
universal and apply to all people in every circumstance,
the mission given to each person is unique because each
person is "one of a kind," and so the details surrounding
the who, what, when, where, why, and how are distinct to
each vocation.

In terms of the rich young man, the Lord responded
to his inquiry with a challenge and invitation: "Jesus said
to him, 'If you would be perfect, go, sell what you possess and give to the poor, and you will have treasure in
heaven; and come, follow me'" (Mt 19:21).

We know from the context of the story that the young
man was "rich" and so this was a very difficult summons
for him. But it would have to be accepted if he was going
to follow the Lord, find his particular vocation, and seek
happiness. Of course, the Bible tells us that the young
man declined the Lord's call.

It would be a mistake to think that the Lord's invitation is only about money. Quite the contrary. The Lord
focused on what was distracting the young man from the
summons. Jesus was calling him to abandon anything

---

6   Ibid., no. 10.

else that claimed an unconditional allegiance from him or that provided him with a false sense of security. He was telling the young man, "Trust me. Leave what is taking you away from me and that is consuming your heart. Come, follow me!"

For the rich young man, it was his money that was absolutized. In moral discernment on end-of-life issues, it could be our sense of autonomy or self will, our desire for independence, a false definition of "quality of life," fear, or an exaggerated anxiety for the future. In all of these, the Lord calls us to abandonment so that we can accept his invitation and "follow him."

In our discernment, we must consider the specific areas of our particular vocation, such as the state of our souls (i.e., are we in grave sin or in an irregular marriage), our duties and responsibilities toward others, our talents and skills, our financial arrangements, our opportunities and authority, and our capabilities and roles in society and in the care of others. Our discernment is never just about us. It always involves our relationship with God and our neighbors.

This point leads us to our third principle. As we approach scenarios that demand decisions, sometimes rapid decisions, we should consider: What is obligatory and what is morally optional? What must I, as a human being and as the one holding this specific vocation, do to inherit eternal life?

Third Principle of Discerning End-of-Life Questions: Obligation or Option

The questions of the rich young man echo in our own hearts, "What must I do to inherent eternal life?" and "What still do I lack?"

As Christian disciples, we desire to do what the Lord asks of us and to do it with trust and joy. Our discernment helps us discover and determine what the best course of care might be in light of the Lord's will for us in each situation. Our discernment, therefore, always addresses a specific state of affairs, in a particular place, and at a specific time.

Relying on the two principles above, our third principle is the distinction between ordinary and extraordinary care. These are the two expressions that are used to clarify what we are called to do.

- *Ordinary* care is that care which is morally *obligatory*.

- *Extraordinary* care is that care which is morally *optional*.

The distinction between the two is essential for our discernment since ordinary care is the summons of the Lord. We are called to abandon all things and to give an obedience of faith to these areas of our end-of-life care. It would be severely regrettable if a person were to have lived their entire life as a faithful Christian but then abandoned the cross and the demands of discipleship at the end of life. In order to prevent this scandal, each of us is obliged to enter into serious discernment, seek counsel, and to do whatever the Lord asks of us.

It's worth remembering again that we do not determine but merely discern what is morally good. Our discernment is marked by our faith in the Lord Jesus and his Church, which is guided by the Holy Spirit. Our first principle stands and is very much needed in this process. It cannot be negotiable; otherwise, we end up following our own fallen preferences.

It's natural to ask, in acknowledging our human vocation and our particular vocation, how we can discern what is ordinary or extraordinary. Is it possible that something is obligatory to one person but not to another? Are these terms applied to specific medical procedures or types of treatment?

The distinction between ordinary and extraordinary care can also be seen as a discernment of benefits and burdens. This means our reflection must involve some practical elements, such as the possibility of survival or benefit to one's person, the degree of possible side effects, the extent of the proposed treatment, our capacity for pain, our responsibilities to other people or society, and our financial means. Within the boundaries set by our first principle, we have to add these other factors into the arena as we decide whether we are obliged to accept treatment or not.

Since our discernment follows our particular vocation, it is possible that a medical procedure or treatment is obligatory for one while optional for another. Following the state of affairs within the boundaries set by our human vocation, we cannot solely identify a specific medical procedure or treatment as ordinary or extraordinary. While the medical community may do so and use the same terms, the Church uses these terms far more holistically and calls for us to consider many areas of our life and not simply the medical invention that is being proposed.

And so our discernment imitates that of the rich young man. We seek to know what the Lord is asking of us and then, like the apostles, to generously respond with trust and confidence in the ways of God. The Lord will never overwhelm us or abandon us. He will only give us what we can carry. But in order to carry what he gives us, we must rely on him and the workings of his grace.

Conclusion

We are the Lord's. As Christian disciples, we follow what Saint Paul called "the more excellent way of love" and we seek, in all that we do, to draw closer to him. In the planning for the end of our lives, and in that difficult process, we must turn closer to the Lord and do all that he asks of us.

The principles above are given so that each of us can search and discover God's will. As Saint Paul also wrote, "Therefore, I urge you, brothers and sisters, in view of God's mercy, to offer your bodies as a living sacrifice, holy and pleasing to God—this is your true and proper worship. Do not conform to the pattern of this world, but be transformed by the renewing of your mind. Then you will be able to test and approve what God's will is—his good, pleasing and perfect will" (Rom 12:1–2).

This is our task as Christians. We must seek to know God's will and not our own. As we surrender our lives to him, let us be brave and also surrender our dying to him as well.

CHAPTER 7

Specific Moral Questions

As I said in the introduction, this chapter consists of rapid questions and answers about specific medical issues that are meant to be quick references and helps to those in pressing situations.

What is the difference between ordinary and extraordinary care?

These two expressions are used to clarify the moral status of any medical treatment or its suspension.

- *Ordinary* care is that care which is morally *obligatory*.

- *Extraordinary* care is that care which is morally *optional*.

The process of identifying whether a particular medical treatment (or its suspension) is ordinary or extraordinary care involves a process of serious discernment. Please see chapter 6 for more detail.

What's the difference between medical care and medical treatment?

The terms "medical treatment" and "medical care" can oftentimes be used interchangeably in popular conversation. But in terms of moral discernment and in directions given to medical personnel, the distinction is critical.

Medical treatment is professionally defined as "the management and care of a patient to combat disease or disorder." This includes, but is not limited to, surgeries, other medical procedures, resuscitation efforts, and the use of prescription drugs.

Medical care is the maintenance of the health and well-being of the patient, as well as efforts to prevent disease, and the general treatment of injuries. Oftentimes, "compassionate measures" are included in this category. These are general efforts to relieve pain and make a patient comfortable.

In conversation with medical personnel, and in drafting advanced directives, the difference between treatment and care must be kept in mind. A person should specify what they want and clarify that, even if medical treatment is suspended, they still want to receive medical care. For example, if a dying patient directs the suspension of all medical attention but then gets the flu, medical personnel would not be able to administer medication. The patient, therefore, might needlessly suffer from a flu that could have been medically treated. This shows us that the clarification between medical treatment and medical care is invaluable.

While most medical personnel would readily offer medical care, the patient or proxy must ensure that they are not blocked from doing so. In general, the distinction between treatment and care can help in navigating the waters of directing what medical attention to approve or suspend and when.

What is meant by the term "informed consent," and why is it important?

Consent is the moral and legal power of a mentally competent patient to decide whether to accept, decline, or delay a medical procedure or treatment. It is called "informed" because medical personnel are required to disclose all benefits and burdens of the procedure or treatment to the patient. This must include all accurate, sufficient, and relevant facts to make a decision. It is classified as "consent" since the final decision belongs to the patient. Such decision-making must be free from any form of coercion, fear mongering, manipulation, or purposeful nondisclosure of pertinent information.

So long as a patient has his cognitive abilities, he holds the power of giving or reserving consent. When a patient has lost his cognitive abilities for whatever reason, the power of giving informed consent rests in a surrogate, also called a medical proxy.

In the process of receiving sufficient information, the believer or patient of goodwill (or his surrogate) should remember his connection to God. He should prudently weigh all options in light of moral truth and assess whether something is ordinary or extraordinary care.

And then, remembering that his life belongs to God, the patient (or proxy) can give his informed consent to whatever will bring about the most good.

What is a medical proxy? How is this person chosen?

A medical proxy, or surrogate, is the person designated by the patient as the one to make his medical decisions if and when he is incapacitated. This designation is usually made through a medical power of attorney that is notarized and/or processed by a lawyer. It is usually kept by the patient, his attorney, the proxy, and/or the patient's primary care doctor.

It is essential that the patient select a proxy who will represent his wishes and worldview, especially in debated issues such as artificial nutrition and hydration. Often, people will instinctually turn to their spouse or eldest child. While this is not necessarily a bad idea, the patient should consider the prospective proxy's moral worldview, psychological temperament, ability to make difficult and life-determining decisions, and his possible financial or temporal gain from the patient's death.

It is important for a patient to understand that if he doesn't select a proxy, then state law will determine one for him. While different states can vary in their laws, the common sequence of possible proxies is: spouse, eldest child, other children by age, oldest sibling, and other siblings by age.

If I'm a medical proxy, am I bound to fulfill any request made by my loved one?

If a loved one asks you to be their medical proxy, it is pivotal that you are clear about his or her desires and discuss his or her moral worldview and wishes. This is important for the prospective patient and will help the proxy make better decisions for unpredicted scenarios. It's also important for you, since you can indicate at that time what your own beliefs are and what you can or cannot consent to in terms of medical care and treatment. This discussion should be revisited on an annual basis as individual's opinions may change with age or with the progression of the illness.

In spite of any possible requests from the patient (or other loved ones), you cannot in any way, or in any situation for any reason, betray moral truth, authentic human dignity, or your own conscience formed on truth. As a Christian believer, *this is a non-negotiable.*

Ideally, any differences that might exist between a medical proxy and a patient would be spelled out beforehand and other arrangements would be made, including the selection of a different or alternate proxy. You should not feel shame or guilt if you have to decline being someone's medical proxy for moral reasons. God's truth takes precedent over even our closest relationships.

What are advanced directives? Are these something I should have?

Advanced directives are a summary of a patient's wishes in various possible and anticipated medical situations. Essentially, it says, "If this happens to me, do this." While such directives can be helpful, they can also be limited and narrow. Since so much of the moral discernment involved in classifying a medical treatment or care as "ordinary" or "extraordinary" is dependent on the unique factors surrounding the case, it is difficult to adequately give directions for them. As bioethicists say, "When you have one situation, you have one situation." Every case is different. It is paramount, therefore, that advanced directives be viewed more as guidelines rather than set directions.

Additionally, not all advanced directives are the same. Some directives are crafted by groups or individuals with agendas that value efficiency over human dignity. Many of these directives dismiss moral truth and goodwill efforts to preserve life. In selecting advanced directives, therefore, it is important that the authors of the respective directives be identified. Moreover, a major battleground issue in advanced directives is the administration of artificial nutrition and hydration. This issue in particular must be evaluated by the patient, and he should be informed about the Church's teachings on it.

While advanced directives have their place and can be helpful within reason, it is more important that a patient's medical proxy know the wishes of the patient, especially as they're contained in advanced directives.

It is vital that a proxy agree with these decisions since oftentimes, especially in an emergency or urgent situation, medical personnel will defer to a medical proxy over advanced directives. Some medical staff see the advanced directives more as a guide to the proxy than to them since they will favor and adhere to a proxy's decisions over advanced directives. Therefore, it's critical that a proxy of one's own worldview and understanding of moral truth be selected with this life-determining role.

What can (or should) I do if my loved one refuses to eat?

It's common for people who are seriously ill or who suffer from dementia to, at some point, stop eating. This can be disturbing to loved ones. The specific actions to be taken will depend on the loved one's health and medical status. For example, if a loved one has a serious (perhaps even terminal) illness but is experiencing a relative degree of stability in terms of normal functioning of their body, but they don't want to eat anymore, then a pastoral or psychological consultation might be needed. It's possible that the person is undergoing some understandable depression. For some, the opportunity to talk about their life, illness, and death outside of family dynamics is enough. This could help them resume a somewhat normal diet. For others, some anti-depressants or anti-anxiety medication might be needed. These steps might also be needed if and when the person needs to receive nutrition and hydration by artificial means.

If a loved one has dementia or is limited in mental capacity, then other measures will be needed. In such a case, clearly communicated and gentle restraints are morally permitted alongside the use of light sedatives so as to either assist the person in eating or to insert a necessary feeding tube.

In either of the above measures, or in others variations of them, it is the responsibility of loved ones (especially the medical proxy) and of medical personnel to ensure that the person who is suffering receives food and hydration. While the person's body can still assimilate them, at no point should food or water (even if artificially administered) ever be suspended or denied to the person who is sick. This includes the aforementioned scenarios where they do not want them or fight against receiving them.

For the Christian believer and for people of goodwill, the option of starving or thirsting someone to death is not an option. The person's autonomy must be tempered in light of moral truth, as well as their medical condition. Even while suffering and lacking the full use of their mental and bodily powers, the person's dignity must be respected and their basic human needs fulfilled.

Medical staff is telling me that artificial nutrition and hydration are extraordinary care. Is this correct?

Food and water are basic human needs, even if provided artificially. Unfortunately, many in the medical community will designate artificial nutrition and hydration as extraordinary care in and of themselves, with no reference to any state of affairs. Contrary to this view, artificially administered food and water are not in them-selves extraordinary care. They are within the realm of basic human care. Giving food or water to another per-son is always a charitable act and one that parallels a basic human need. Only in situations when the body is unable to assimilate them (or they become harmful to the patient) are artificially administered food and water classified as extraordinary care and properly suspended.

We can imagine our reaction, or the reaction of any Christian or person of goodwill, if someone were to refuse to change a terminally ill person's adult diaper or bedding because "they're going to die anyway." We would rightly be appalled. We expect that these basic human services would be provided until the person actually dies. In a similar way, this is how moral truth approaches food and water. It's a service that is not negotiable so long as the person's body can receive and benefit from the food and water, even if these are given artificially.

The fact that a person is unable to feed himself or drink water himself and must, therefore, be provided these basic human needs artificially does not—in any way—preclude medical professionals or family members from providing this basic care to the patient.

Since they are a part of basic human care, when is it possible to suspend nutrition and hydration?

Every human person has dignity and a human voca-tion, a call to live and cherish our shared humanity. This acknowledgment of human dignity, and of our solidar-ity as human beings with one another, demands that we generously provide basic human care, which includes food and water (even if administered artificially). If we stopped these basic needs, then we are starving or dehydrating the person to death. This would be euthanasia since it is the deprivation of food and water that are causing death rather than the person's illness or medical condition.

The only time that food and hydration can be suspended is when a person's body is unable to assimilate them and/or they cause harm to the person. In these cases, the good offered by food and water would not actually be serving any good and so they must be suspended. In these cases, this would not be euthanasia since the person's medical condition is causing death and not the suspension of food and water.

This last point must be emphasized. In the discernment of when to suspend nutrition and hydration (even if artificially administered), the rule of thumb is the pressing question: *What will cause the death of this person?* If death occurs because of the removal of food and water, then it is euthanasia. If, however, death is caused by the person's medical condition or illness, then it is not euthanasia (even if food and water had to be suspended toward the end of life because of the illness and the inability of the body to assimilate them).

What should I do if medical personnel put pressure on me to accept treatment or care that's not morally acceptable or withhold necessary treatment?

The majority of people in the medical profession are there because they sincerely wish to help people, and so we should always seek to approach them with respect and appropriate deference. At times, however, certain medical professionals overstep appropriate bounds and apply improper pressure to patients, medical proxies, and families.

The intentions behind such unseemly behavior are diverse. For some medical personnel, they are raw utilitarians and disregard spiritual or religious considerations. They can become impatient and dismissive to patients or proxies who try to explain their discernment of the person's dignity beyond just their abilities or functions. For other medical personnel, they might be open to spiritual considerations but have no developed understanding of Catholic teaching and the reasons behind it. This could even include some Catholic medical professionals who do not know their faith as well as they know their medical practice.

Regardless of the reasons, the Christian patient or proxy must be steadfast. In the face of possible condescension, disparaging comments, and pressure, we are called to be advocates who can provide answers with explanations, apply our answers to the medical options presented, and ask the medical personnel to respect both our beliefs and our decisions.

If medical personnel continue to put pressure on a patient or proxy, they should request to see a patient advocate and/or ask to have a different doctor. A patient advocate is a hospital official who helps negotiate troubles between families and medical staff.

No one, especially someone who is sick or emotionally distressed, should be taken advantage of and have their beliefs and decisions derided or dismissed. Medical professionals are in service to the sick, and they should always revere the decisions of their patients (and proxies), especially when their decisions are based on holistic reasons such as their spiritual or religious worldview. Additionally, any patient or proxy can request to see a Catholic priest who can clarify our teachings and give support to the Catholic party.

Is a breathing tube extraordinary care?

This is a good question because it presents an opportunity to clarify an essential point in the moral discernment between whether a medical procedure or care is ordinary or extraordinary.

In the medical community, these designations are made about the treatments or procedures themselves. And so, a doctor might just say, "Yes, a breathing tube is extraordinary care." In terms of moral discernment, however, we wouldn't just say that in a vacuum. In order to make any moral decision, we need more information; namely, the patient's unique state of affairs. This additional insight is critical since a breathing tube could be ordinary care in one instance while extraordinary in another. For example, for someone of severe old age who is dying of cancer, the breathing tube could be extraordinary. For an infant whose lungs need some help breathing, it would certainly be ordinary. It's the same breathing tube, but the state of affairs gives it a different moral status.

The distinction between ordinary care (which is morally binding on our consciences) and extraordinary care (which is morally optional) is made through the interaction of several key factors, such as the current health of the patient, the seriousness of the procedure, the rate of success, the spiritual standing of the person with God, the patient's temperament and capacity to endure pain, the patient's vocation and responsibilities to loved ones or to the community, et cetera (please see chapter 6 for more details). Only through all these factors could a responsible and holistic designation be made about the moral status of a breathing tube.

With the above points made, it's also very important to indicate that there is more flexibility with a breathing tube than a feeding tube.

How is a breathing tube morally different from a feeding tube?

While often popularly seen as two sides of the same coin, there is a fundamental difference between the two. The breathing tube is seen within the general realm of extraordinary care since it's an external help to the body. This doesn't mean a breathing tube is always extraordinary, but the conditions are broader for its application in this moral designation.

The feeding tube, however, is not considered a medical procedure at all since it's a direct act of kindness by loved ones (even if administered artificially) and is assimilated by the body. It becomes an internal part of the body. For these reasons, the feeding tube is not placed within the designations of ordinary and extraordinary care but within the stricter realm of basic human care. This designation emphasizes the importance of the feeding tube and indicates that the conditions surrounding when it can (and cannot) be removed are much stricter since it pertains to the immediate care of the person.

It seems there are so many medical measures to stay alive. How do I know "when to say when"?

It's true that contemporary Western medicine has taken us to new heights. With these developments, we have the odd but sincere question: when is it okay to die?

Any answer to this question should be grounded on a strong respect for our dignity as children of God and by a desire for heaven. The consoling truth is that God knows the moment of our conception and the moment of our death. Of course, this begs the question again: if God knows the date of our death, how are we to know when to say when?

First, we need to have a strong understanding of ordinary and extraordinary care. When is something obligatory and when is it optional (again, please see chapter 6 for more information)? If something is ordinary care, then we must accept it. If something is extraordinary care, then we have the moral option of accepting or declining.

In such cases, it is permissible to decline a medical procedure or treatment, even if it means we might die by not accepting it. In such a case, we can say "when" and let a natural death play itself out.

Incidentally, it's a noble and beautiful thing to pray for a holy death and to peacefully accept death when it comes. Of course, such aspirations must always follow moral truth and be surrounded by a strong conviction of the goodness and dignity of human life. We can desire death because life has become difficult or we want to avoid suffering at all cost. This is an intention that can cause an otherwise virtuous desire to become less noble and even sinful.

If I don't approve of a medical treatment, isn't that euthanasia?

Before answering this, we should make sure we understand what euthanasia is. Euthanasia is the taking of a seriously ill person's life by a willful act or omission. The denial of medical treatment can be euthanasia in some cases, but not in others. The difference is found in the distinction between ordinary and extraordinary care. In cases of ordinary care, which is always morally obligatory, then any suspension or refusal of medical treatment is euthanasia. In cases of extraordinary care, which is morally optional care, medical treatment can be denied or suspended, and the intention of the patient or proxy is also a deciding factor. In such cases, there's a process of discernment, which always respects moral truth and our dignity as human beings, by which a patient or proxy comes to the decision that something is within the bounds of extraordinary care.

In such a situation, a person (or proxy) can morally pass or suspend treatment. The person or proxy is choosing here to avoid morally optional care. The decision is not motivated by a hatred of life, a denunciation of life's goodness, or a dismissal or redefinition of human dignity. The decision recognizes the blessedness of life and cherishes and honors it but also realizes that the optional care would serve no good (and might actually cause harm). And so, the decision in this case chooses to allow a natural death to play itself out. In spiritual terms, it reflects the prayer of Simeon in the New Testament: "Lord, now you let your servant go in peace; your word has been fulfilled" (Lk 2:29).

In some situations, the actual act or omission of euthanasia can be the exact same act or omission that is done in cases of morally optional care that is denied or suspended. In such scenarios, the moral difference is precisely the intention of the patient or proxy.

If a patient or proxy just wants to "end it," denouncing life and seeing it as a curse, and so wants to die, then this intention can make the act or omission (which could objectively be morally optional) into an act of euthanasia. A proper and life-affirming intention, even in the midst of pain and suffering, is needed alongside an act of extraordinary care.

And so the designation of the act or omission as ordinary and extraordinary, as well as the intention of the patient or proxy in extraordinary circumstances, are the deciding factors of whether an act is one of euthanasia or not.

What is a DNR?

The acronym DNR stands for "do not resuscitate." This is a directive by a person that in the case of imminent death (usually from a sudden attack to a person's heart, brain, or other vital organ), no extraordinary means are to be used. For example, if someone is undergoing cardiac arrest, there is to be no CPR done and/or no use of an automated external defibrillator (AED). The person is to be left alone and the attack allowed to play out so that a natural death ensues.

Whenever we approach end-of-life questions, we should always be attentive and sensitive to details and to the temperament of the one who's suffering. Some people who love life and see it as a blessing are still unable to endure the psychological or physical sufferings of a long-term illness, one that is intensified by a sudden attack or by debilitations that might be caused by a sudden attack to their otherwise good health. In light of these and other considerations, it is morally acceptable to choose a DNR. In choosing it, however, our intention must be one that values our life, even as we give direction for our lives not to be resuscitated so that a natural death can occur.

To clarify, this would not be euthanasia but a decision not to accept extraordinary care (which is always morally optional) so that a natural death can happen.

In discerning a DNR, an individual must be careful to guard against malicious intentions, such as, "I don't want to live that way or with this suffering," or, "My life has no value with this suffering and so I'm going to end it." Such intentions are anti-life and should be foreign to Christian believers and to people of goodwill. Incidentally, this darker intention could change an otherwise good act into one that is akin to euthanasia.

As a point of clarification, it should be pointed out that these darker intentions are radically different from the intention of the person who honors their life and is sincerely unable to live with the debilitations that could be caused by sudden attacks to their health.

With that said, if we are a medical proxy and our loved one has chosen a DNR, then we must always assume the best intention and ensure that the DNR is respected by medical personnel.

How much pain medication can be given?

As a general rule of thumb, the amount of pain medication that can be given should match the level of pain and allow a person to rest comfortably. There should be caution not to needlessly over-medicate someone, especially if it means the unnecessary loss of their mental capacities. On the other hand, pain medication should not be refused to a patient who has an authentic medical need for it. The dose and administering of the pain medicine should be monitored and reduced or stopped when the pain or discomfort has stopped.

It should be pointed out that some patients may choose to wait to receive pain medication because they want to remain mentally sharp, or wish to offer up their sufferings, and/or they desire additional unencumbered quality time with loved ones. In such a case, the wish of the patient in this circumstance must be respected. On the other hand, the choice to offer up suffering is not for another person to make. We do not know the level of pain that a person is enduring. If they ask for an appropriate level of pain medication, it must be given to them. No one else can impose or add a noble or sanctifying intention to another's sufferings.

What if pain medication ends up taking a person's life? Is that euthanasia?

If someone gives an intentional and purposeful overdose of pain medication to a suffering person with the hope of ending life, then the act is clearly euthanasia.

But most people do not fall in the scenario just described. Most people have goodwill and want to do the right thing and make sure their loved one isn't suffering. Here's a helpful principle for such situations: the level of pain medication can be given to match the level of a person's pain.

In applying this principle to people who are suffering intensely, it may happen that the pain medication will cause the loss of mental capacity and hasten the person's death. In such a case, the deciding factor for the moral status of the person or proxy's action is whether the intention was to either take life or solely lessen pain, even if there was the foreseeable but unintended consequence of the loss of life.

If the intention was to solely relieve pain and these efforts actually caused the hastening of death, then the act is within moral truth. There is no guilt. The reason why is because the pain medication did not cause the person's death; his initial illness or disease caused his death. The pain medication attempted to treat the pain caused by the illness or disease and in that effort *unintentionally* hastened the person's death.

If the intention in giving the pain medication, however, was to take life, then it becomes an act of euthanasia. It violates clear boundaries of moral truth. There is guilt since the intention was to cause death with the pain medication.

In distinguishing between the two possibilities, it's important to emphasize the focus of moral truth, which is to both honor the person's dignity and to proportionately relieve his pain.

If my loved one is in a coma or a PVS (persistent vegetative state), am I able to suspend nutrition and hydration?

If a loved one is in a persistent vegetative state (PVS) or a coma of any form, then nutrition and hydration cannot be suspended so long as their body is able to assimilate and process it. The reason for this is that a person in a PVS or coma is not dying. This is not an end-of-life question. The person is alive but in a different state. Incidentally, the term "vegetative" is a medical one and should not give the impression that somehow the person is less human or that any of their human dignity has been diminished. They are fully human and have all the rights of every other human person. As such, they deserve and are to be given all aspects of basic human care, which includes food and drink, even if given artificially.

There is immense pressure to euthanize people in a PVS, but the Christian believer is called to see the person's dignity and worth even in the midst of their condition and to protect and care for them.

What help is there if I'm really afraid of dying?

As human beings with the power of reason, we can know and reflect on the reality of our own deaths. This awareness is heightened when we're up against a serious medical situation or illness. It becomes reality when we are terminally ill or in the dying process.

Since self-preservation is one of our most basic drives, it is common for anyone (even a person of faith) to have a natural fear of dying. The reality of concluding our life in this world, and of saying goodbye to our loved ones and to the life we've become accustomed to, certainly brings up some anxiety and fear in minds and hearts.

For the unbeliever, he is left with such restlessness. For the Christian, however, there is an answer to this trepidation and uneasiness. The believer turns to the Paschal Mystery, which is the passion, death, and resurrection of Jesus Christ.

In the Paschal Mystery, the Christian offers up his fear as a gift to the Lord Jesus and unites it to the Lord's own sufferings. In this way, his emotional suffering becomes redemptive and brings about a greater good in his life and in the lives of others. As holy ones have said through-out the ages, "There is nothing worse in this world than wasted suffering." The Christian, therefore, knows the power of his suffering and offers it up for his good and the good of those in need.

The Christian also reminds himself, and asks fellow believers to remind him, that death has lost its sting. The Lord Jesus has destroyed the kingdom of sin and death by the power of his resurrection. The Lord offers each of us a share in his glory. As we suffer and are distressed over the prospect of our own deaths, we are consoled in the sure knowledge that this life leads to another. As we pray in the funeral Mass, "Indeed, Lord, for your faith-ful, life is changed, not ended." This is the hope that has been given to us in Jesus Christ. In dark moments, when fear wants to overwhelm us, we can claim the light of the Resurrection and find a renewed peace and calm in that wonderful mystery.

As a help to strengthening our faith in the Resurrection, we can pray the Glorious Mysteries of the Rosary and read (or have read to us) the different Passion and Resurrection accounts in the Gospel books. Additionally, the praying of the Psalms in the Old Testament can bring spiritual encouragement and consolation.

By fanning into flame the graces of the Resurrection, the Christian finds a supernatural readiness and bold-ness for death. The believer knows that another chapter (this one, final and eternal) awaits him beyond death. And so while the Christian might have a natural fear of death and dying, it is elevated and transformed by the Resurrection.

In addition to the above mentioned spiritual practices, the Christian tradition has also recommended and endorsed prayers to Saint Joseph for a happy death. Since Saint Joseph died with the Blessed Virgin Mary on one side of him and the Lord Jesus on the other, he is the best patron for a holy and peaceful death. There are many prayers written to Saint Joseph in this spirit. Here's one that's very popular:

> O Blessed Joseph, who died in the arms of Jesus and Mary, obtain for me, I beseech you, the grace of a happy death.
>
> In that hour of dread and anguish, assist me by your presence, and protect me by your power against the enemies of my salvation.
>
> Into your sacred hands, living and dying, Jesus, Mary, Joseph, I commend my soul. Amen.

How do I handle the guilt of making a decision that ended a person's life?

First, to be fair, the intensity, sleep deprivation, confusion, and anxiety of being a proxy cannot be underestimated. Oftentimes, after his or her loved one's death, it could take weeks to catch up on sleep and regain his or her bearings. And, of course, hind sight is 20/20.

If in discerning and reviewing the decisions it's realized that a morally bad decision was made, the proxy should seek out a priest and ask for guidance and possibly the sacrament of Reconciliation.

If, however, the proxy can acknowledge that all the decisions were within moral boundaries, even though death occurred, then any "guilt" they feel has to be rejected because it is not founded on moral truth.

Spiritual theology helps us understand that the soul's experience of guilt and grief are felt in the same way. And so a person can be grieving but think that they are in a process of guilt. It takes the intellect to identify and help the person to realize the source of their sorrow. In morally sound cases, it is most likely grief that is causing the sorrow. The person is grieving the loss of their loved one. They are mourning. By recognizing the real experience that their soul is undergoing, proxies can avoid needless perceived guilt and can begin the healing process by acknowledging their grief and letting themselves grieve their loss.

Therefore, examine your conscience. Name whatever happened in the care of your loved one, and then take the proper course of action so that you can be free and begin the healing process.

CHAPTER 8

The Catholic Funeral

For the Dead

Some time ago, I was approached by a well-intentioned, non-Catholic funeral director. He wanted to add certain things to the funeral Mass that are outside of the Catholic tradition. I declined his requests. When I attempted to explain why these additions were not possible, the gentleman interrupted me and asserted, "Reverend, I understand, but the funeral is for the living."

It was an awkward moment, especially when I replied, "No, the funeral is for the dead."

The man was speechless. While he was quiet, I went on and elaborated that for Catholics, the funeral is primarily an offering of prayers, and of the Eucharist, for the repose of the deceased Christian's soul. And only then, after this principal spiritual duty is given attention, does the funeral provide the deceased person's loved ones needed consolation and the strength of grace.

The encounter above exposes a lot of assumptions and some misunderstandings about the Catholic funeral. These misunderstandings are true not only among our non-Catholic neighbors but also among the Catholic faithful in the Church.

In light of this observation, some questions need to be asked: What is a Catholic funeral? How is it unique among other burial ceremonies and celebrations of life of non-Catholics? Why is the Catholic funeral significant?

The Purpose of the Catholic Funeral

The Catholic funeral is the solemn prayer and supplication of the Church on earth, as a portion of the Body of Christ. It seeks the mercy of God and eternal rest and peace for its member who has experienced temporal death.

In Christ, the funeral's purpose is to assist in the Christian's transition from this life to the next: from the Church on earth, possibly through the Church in purgatory, and then hopefully to the Church eternal in heaven.

As the Body of Christ, we pray that the Christian will rest in Abraham's bosom and know the joys of paradise forever. The family and loved ones of the deceased Christian have a special place in this prayerful action of the whole church. While this special place is a favored participation in the communal prayer of the whole body, it does not of itself define or shape the prayer.

The Funeral Stations

The funeral is best understood as a process of three stations that are meant to order and guide both the prayer for the dead and the grief and sorrow of the loved ones.

The first station is called the vigil, popularly known as the wake, and was traditionally celebrated in the family home. Perhaps celebrated in a funeral parlor now, it is still a casual and deeply family-centered time of prayer and is meant as an opportunity for eulogies, stories, and common sharing. The vigil begins the liturgical prayer for the deceased Christian.

The second station, and the central act of the Body of Christ, is the Mass of Christian Burial; what most people think of as the funeral. There is an option for this prayer to be celebrated outside of Mass, but it is only to be used for serious pastoral reasons because of the power of the Eucharist in assisting the repose of the soul. This station has the Eucharistic offering as the heart, and it is the focus of the entire funeral process.

The Mass expands the prayer of the family and places it within the overall prayer of the universal Body of Christ. The family is now a member and participates in the sacrifice for the deceased with all their brothers and sisters in Christ.

For this reason, the family, loved ones, funeral directors, or even priests cannot alter or change, modify or accommodate the Mass to any personal or esoteric desires. Eulogies are not preferred because the focus is on the resurrection and the person's eternal life.

The music for the funeral is to be from within the church's tradition and not from popular fads or cultural trends, even if favored by the deceased. Photo displays, ostentatious flower arrangements, or anything that might take away from the focus of the Mass is to be tempered or removed.

This is the prayer of the Church and not of any one person, family, or congregation. It is meant to unite the whole body and serve the deceased person.

The third station is the rite of committal, commonly called the graveside service. This is when the Church accompanies the family to the place of burial, blesses the place of rest, and offers further prayers for the deceased Christian.

Conclusion

The Catholic funeral process is a time of intercession and supplication. Through these traditional ritual acts, God's grace is given, the departed Christian receives help, and loved ones can find consolation.

The funeral is for the departed, and that emphasis should not be lost. In general, the supernatural focus and ancient beauty of the Catholic funeral must be cherished and preserved at all costs. The spiritual opportunity offered by it should be eagerly sought out by the family and loved ones of the departed Christian and should be beautifully celebrated and prayed by the local parish community.

CHAPTER 9

Prayers for the Dead

Why Prayers for the Dead?

People are often curious or shocked when they encounter the Catholic custom of praying for the dead. They ask, "Why do you pray for them? They're dead!"

The question reflects some strongly held cultural beliefs about death: it is a final end, we're permanently separated from loved ones, and there's nothing else beyond death. As Catholics, we assent to none of these convictions. In our lives, we hold up a vastly different creed. And this creed is grounded and inspired by the resurrection of the Lord Jesus from the dead.

The Body of Christ

Our central belief, which unites and gives expression to other beliefs, is that all believers—in varying degrees—are one body in Jesus Christ. This body is invigorated by the Holy Spirit, and nothing—not even death—can divide the body. As Saint Paul teaches us, "For as in one body we have many members, and all the members do not have the same function, so we, though many, are one body in Christ, and individually members one of another" (Rom 12:4–5).

As members of the body of Christ, therefore, we each have certain blessings and graces. We also have particular opportunities and responsibilities as believers. One of these sacred privileges is praying for one another, and this duty does not end at temporal death.

In this life on earth, I frequently ask my fellow believers and friends to pray for me, to make intercession for my needs and situations. Likewise, others ask for my prayers and I show my love and concern by making supplication for them. Within the body of Christ, this causes no barrier or problems with our relationship to Jesus but actually expands and deepens it.

Death has no power over this prayerful opportunity won by the Lord Jesus's resurrection from the dead and the continual activity of the Holy Spirit.

The Lord's Example

In his public ministry, Jesus quoted the Old Testament and identified God with Abraham, Isaac, and Jacob. He asserted, "God is not the God of the dead, but of the living" (Mt 22:32). The patriarchs of old live on in eternity, and Jesus points to them as witnesses to us of everlasting life. We seek their help on earth.

Within the body of Christ, we turn to all the saints, the friends of God, who are our older brothers and sisters in heaven. From them, we still ask for guidance, encouragement, and prayer.

Purgatory

As believers, we also remember our loved ones and fellow believers who have left this world marked with the sign of faith. We pray that the Lord will be merciful in his judgment.

Certainly, the faith community hopes that all its members find their way to heaven after death, but some souls aren't quite ready. They need some additional purgation, or purifying work by God's grace, in order to make them fit for paradise.

Perhaps the believer died with sin on his soul, or there was a habit of sin or an offense to others that caused deep harm, and so the soul carries some temporal punishment that needs to be cleansed by Jesus Christ in order to enter heaven without any stain or entanglement with darkness.

Traditionally, this state of purification is called purgatory. In this case, the name truly says it all. Just as Jesus Christ *purges* and cleanses human souls in this life, and other believers can assist and serve as instruments by which this saving work is accomplished, so believers are welcomed and obliged to continue their help in this redemptive mission to those souls in purgatory.

As in this life, so in the next. Every Christian can still be a means through which God's grace works and from which others can be saved by Jesus Christ.

And so Christians offer supplication for the dead because they love them and are still a part of them in Jesus Christ. Their prayers work and are a sign of the service and fellowship they hold with them in the Resurrection.

The believer's petition is offered because she wants her beloved dead to enter paradise and share in the Lord's glory.

Conclusion

In Christ, therefore, we are all one body. Death comes and death goes. In Jesus Christ, we are born to eternal life and have everlasting communion with one another in him.

We see this communion of all the holy ones in Jesus Christ in our tradition of prayers, in the way we celebrate the Mass, and in the hope that surrounds us as Christian believers.

CHAPTER 10

Our Takeaway

Source of Hope

For the Christian believer, the accounts of the passion, death, and resurrection of Jesus Christ are full of wisdom for life, a happy death, and an eternal worldview. Within the sacred accounts of the sufferings and glory of Jesus Christ, we find the inspiration and hope that are needed to live our lives well in this world and so prepare ourselves in Jesus Christ for an everlasting life in heaven.

From these pages, therefore, we should draw two accounts as we close this book.

As We Suffer

As we suffer, we should recall the Lord and his immense suffering throughout the Passion, especially as it begins in the Garden of Gethsemane. With sorrow in his heart and blood flowing from his pores, the Lord asked God, "Father, let this cup pass." This simple but profound prayer is oftentimes, in one form or another, the petition of those who are sick and suffering.

Lord, please let the cancer be gone. Lord, please let me wake up after this surgery. Lord, please let me make it to my daughter's wedding.

And similar supplications abound throughout the body of believers around the world. We ask for consolation and healing. We ask for more time. We ask for some control over what's going to happen.

The Lord Jesus, however, wasn't done with his prayer. He prays, "Father, if you are willing, let this cup pass. But not my will, your will be done" (cf. Lk 22:42). In the throes of his overwhelming pain, Jesus surrendered his life and desires to God the Father.

In this way, he serves as a model for how we should approach our own sufferings, sorrows, and distress. The Lord shows us how to live in a spirit of abandonment to God's divine providence and his loving care for each of us. It's never easy or comfortable, but God sends his grace and his angels to help us. When we are sick and have no control, we are invited to turn to the Lord. We are summoned to be with him in Gethsemane and to offer our sufferings as a gift with his own sufferings.

As We Accompany the Suffering

As we accompany those who suffer, either as a medical proxy or as a loved one, we suffer as well. As we see the person we love (and who loves us) in soreness, distress, and pain, we too are beside ourselves. We also are in agony as we feel the helplessness and vulnerability of the situation. At times, we don't know what to do; many times, there isn't anything we can do.

With such a state of affairs, we can turn again to the Passion narratives of the Gospels. In the sacred account, we see two figures. First, there's Simon of Cyrene. Second, there is Mary of Nazareth.

In the Passion account, Simon of Cyrene helps the Lord to carry his cross. There isn't much more he can do. With crowds yelling and guards pushing, Simon is simply there and helps to carry a portion of the weight. There wasn't much to say and there weren't any warm feelings. Simon was there and he carried some of the weight.

In our own accompaniment, Simon can help us. At times, we think we need to have great wisdom for our loved one. Other times, we think we're supposed to fix something or there are expectations of us. In the end, however, Simon reminds us that just being there and helping—even with just a small portion of the burden— is enough. Most of the times, we just need to be there, love generously, wait patiently, and do whatever small thing might be asked of us. We might want to cure heart disease, but our loved one just wants a cup of water.

Also in the Passion narrative, we see Mary of Nazareth. The presence of the Lord's mother is a moving one. As his heart was torn and his body was beaten, so was hers. And yet she said nothing. She imposed nothing. Mary was there. She prayed. She loved. She was, and is always, the *stabat mater*—the standing mother.

Our Lady is strong for her Son. She is there for her Son. She is a servant to the cross and will become a witness to the resurrection of her Son!

And Mary is here for us. She is praying for us as we imitate her at the Calvary—the bedside or in the hospital room—of our own loved ones. Not knowing what to do or what to say, we are called to imitate the *stabat mater*. We are called to be there. To pray and to love.

In our own brokenness and vulnerability, as we take on a portion of our own loved one's sufferings, we are not alone. Our Lady is with us. She is showing us what to do. And we are called to do our best.

We Once Were

The path of suffering and the journey of walking with those who suffer is one that points us to the reality of our own deaths and opens up for us a reflection on eternity. As we go through these different endeavors, we cannot miss the grace and wisdom that abounds throughout them.

Our task is to stay focused on Jesus Christ and the promises of his resurrection. As we go through the sufferings and anxieties of this life, our hope is in Jesus Christ.

We have been born. We live. We die as we have lived. We have the potential in Jesus Christ to live forever. What will we do?

Let the words of some noble Capuchin Franciscans friars, which are contained in the famous "Bone Chapel" of the Immaculate Conception Church in Rome, speak to us today:

> *What you are, we once were;*
> *What we are, you will one day be.*